Cauê Vazquez La Scala Teixeira

Advanced training techniques for

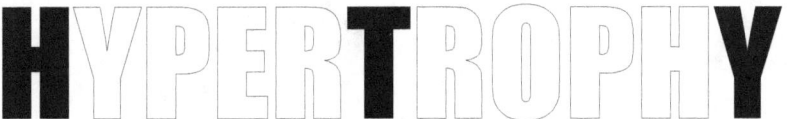

2nd Edition – Updated and Expanded

CreateSpace

2016

Citation:
Teixeira, CVLS. Advanced training techniques for hypertrophy. 2nd ed.
CreateSpace, 2016.

Bibliography
ISBN: 978-1532889462

Cover design: Paulo Henrique Farias – Publicist and Designer

I dedicate this book to all those who contributed or contribute, directly or indirectly, consciously or unconsciously, to my professional development and constant search for excellence. In particular, to my parents, grandparents, brother, wife, and son. You are my inspiration.

PRESENTATION

I am a declared lover of weight training and my relationship with this modality started early, more precisely during adolescence. At that time, my objective was to become "big" and I thought nothing was better than weight training for me to achieve muscle hypertrophy.

I started to train long before I became a Physical Education professional and at first I looked for information in training magazines, bodybuilders' videos, and in the experience of older people and of training partners. I must say that this experience was useful to me.

However, when entering the university and facing a barrage of technical and scientific information, my critical sense surfaced and I developed a highly questioning spirit.

Since then, I started to retrieve all my previous experiences in weight training and to compare them to what I was learning every day. I realized that beliefs and empiricism had been my faithful companions until then, ranging from the manipulation of the simplest variables to "adventures" with food supplements.

However, among all the responses I was receiving from science, I realized that something still needed to be investigated, i.e., the famous advanced training techniques.

Those "crazy" combinations that we copied or invented in the gym to wear down the muscles and make them grow were totally empirical and little was known about their physiological aspects and their supposed superiority over the conventional model.

However, a little more than one decade ago considerable scientific advances permitted a better understanding of the effects of different training techniques on muscle hypertrophy. What was missing was an account that would synthesize this information in a clear manner in order to facilitate access by the general public devoted to weight training. But this is no longer missing!

In this book I provide information about advanced weight training techniques, exploring forms of execution and specifically analyzing their effects on muscle hypertrophy (and related factors). I hope that, with the information presented here, the techniques can be applied in a more intelligent and productive manner.

I wish to emphasize that in no way do the readings and investigations about this topic end here. So, may this book serve to encourage new and more in-depth studies.

Good reading!

PREFACE

I always like to say that Science without practical application is incomplete and that practice without the backing of Science may be incorrect. Thus, I am happy and honored by the invitation to write a Preface to the book Advanced Training Techniques for Hypertrophy.

Over decades of systematic strength training, coaches, athletes and sports scientists have looked for training strategies that can potentiate the stimulation of loads, permitting positive adjustments and enhancing the results, also for more trained subjects. Thus, dozens of so-called advanced training techniques for muscle hypertrophy have been proposed. The book describes how these techniques are applied, highlighting their objectives and when to use them for the structuring of the training process – periodization. In addition, the book has a theoretical foundation based on scientific evidence for the techniques that have already been investigated in published scientific articles. Regarding the author, Cauê La Scala Teixeira, I have witnessed his professional evolution from graduation to the present day, his constant search for improvement and updating, while being open to discussion and suggestions. Furthermore, I have witnessed the practical experience he has acquired since his adolescence, when he started to practice weight training at the same gym, the Sparta Halteres Clube, where I worked out. Finally, I wish to say that I feel greatly rewarded when the author thanks me for my participation in his professional development. Thank you, Cauê!

As for you, reader, enjoy the book! I guarantee an excellent reading.

Prof. Dilmar Pinto Guedes Júnior, M.Sc

CONTENTS

Introduction, 11

Chapter 1. Biological principles of training, 15

    Principle of progressive overload, 15

    Principle of variability, 16

    Principle of biological individuality, 17

Chapter 2. Muscle hypertrophy, 19

    Mechanical tension, 20

    Metabolic stress, 22

Chapter 3. Advanced training techniques, 25

    Techniques that emphasize mechanical tension, 27

    Techniques that emphasize metabolic stress, 32

    Mixed techniques, 42

    Undefined techniques, 55

Final considerations, 63

References, 65

About the author, 73

INTRODUCTION

The practice of weight training is surrounded by cultural beliefs and aspects that serve as paradigms for training prescription due to the fact that the science related to physical exercise took time to explore the understanding of resistance exercises. In past decades, researchers have devoted time and money almost exclusively to scientific research designed to understand the adaptations resulting from aerobic exercises, which contributed to the fact that they have long been considered the main exercises for health promotion in humans.

However, at that time, despite the lack of scientific evidence, weight training enthusiasts already knew that resistance exercises promote adaptations that aerobic training could not induce at the same proportions. The most evident example is the increase in strength and muscle mass. These enthusiasts also noted that, if they maintained the training routines for long periods of time without major modifications, the organic responses tended to stabilize or even to regress. Within this context, there is the legendary Canadian figure Joe Weider, who was one of the pioneers of bodybuilding. At the end of the 1930s, Joe was responsible for systematizing a training model aimed at increasing muscle mass (hypertrophy) and for popularizing what was known at the time as bodybuilding.

With strong empirical support, given that the science related to exercise, especially resistance exercise, was in its infancy, Joe and his contemporaries created many of the techniques that we know and practice until today in bodybuilding. The objective of those techniques was to permit variations in physical and motivational stimuli in order to prevent/break plateaus both in performance and in the readiness to train. However, research on resistance exercise has grown substantially in recent decades and, although further evidence is still needed, many aspects related to weight training techniques have been investigated and clarified. Nevertheless, empiricism is still strong among weight lifting practitioners, which even today causes us to live with situations such as those mentioned below:

- "My friend trained that way and it worked. I will train so too!"
- "I watched the training of the current Mr. Olympia on the internet. If I train the same way, I shall become like him!'
- "I saw the training of an actress and model in a magazine. The results were great. I will copy it!"

After the recognition of Physical Education by the health area almost two decades ago, the visibility of Physical Education professionals and, consequently, their responsibility has grown. As a consequence, a scientific approach to this field also increased and many practices that before were empirically based started to be investigated.

In this scenario, the different training techniques for hypertrophy have raised the interest of researchers in the area of resistance exercise and the scientific production related to this topic has increased. Today, although several factors still need to be elucidated, considerable advances have been made in the understanding of the physiological effects of different training techniques.

Therefore, the objective of this book is to explore the technical and scientific details of advanced weight training techniques based on the comprehensive practical experience of the author as a practitioner and coach, associated with the most recent and relevant scientific findings on this topic. The approach is directed at muscle hypertrophy. It should be emphasized that the idea is not to exhaust the topic, given that the number of scientific articles available in the literature on the techniques reported is small and many other methods have not yet been investigated. Thus, the aim is to sum up current knowledge and to encourage new studies.

I wish the reader an excellent use of the material. Good reading and great training!

CHAPTER 1
Biological principles of training

The biological principles of training have long been reported in the specialized literature. These principles serve as a guide for the prescription of any type of physical training since they are linked to the biological and physiological characteristics of humans.

When we refer to training directed at advanced weight training practitioners, the understanding of some principles becomes even more important. This chapter will discuss the principles that are most relevant for the prescription of training directed at these practitioners.

Principle of progressive overload

According to this principle, the occurrence of adaptation in the body requires a previous stimulus that disturbs its state of dynamic equilibrium, referred to by some as homeostasis. In response to this disturbance, the body sets off a series of reactions aimed at reestablishing the state of dynamic equilibrium (Teixeira and Guedes Jr., 2009).

In physical training, these disturbances are called overload. This overload provides levels of stress that disturb homeostasis. After the stimulus, when the body is submitted to appropriate rest and nutrition, homeostasis is reestablished and the levels of physical fitness rise (overcompensation) (Teixeira and Guedes Jr., 2009; 2013). However, with time the body will become less responsive to overload and the latter thus needs to be increased gradually so that the stress continues to stimulate progressive adaptations.

Principle of variability

Stimuli of similar magnitudes, if maintained for a long period of time, do no longer provide continuous adaptations of the body. In addition, there is the risk of reversal of the adaptations if the periods of stimulus maintenance are extremely prolonged. This is called continuity/reversibility (Pereira and Souza Jr., 2005).

This biological characteristic supports the need for constant stimulus variation by manipulating the volume and, especially, the intensity of training. This necessity becomes more evident in experienced practitioners (Teixeira and Guedes Jr., 2009).

Several studies in the area of periodized training state that a higher frequency of stimulus variation can be an important factor to potentiate the results. In this respect, daily undulatory periodization models have been shown to be highly effective (Minozzo et al., 2008; Fleck, 2011). Thus, the alternation of training sessions that do not only explore different techniques, but especially different stimuli (tension, metabolic or mixed stimuli; see Chapter 3), may be an interesting strategy to provide constant hypertrophic adaptations.

Principle of biological individuality

Every human being is unique and responds uniquely to different stimuli. Thus, the same stimuli may elicit different adaptations in two different organisms (Pereira and Souza Jr., 2005).

Consequently, no scientific publication replaces individual evaluations of the practitioner. Science should serve as a guide, but does not guarantee that the results observed in the studies are 100% reproducible across the population.

The physical conditions of the practitioner should therefore be evaluated and reevaluated with certain periodicity in order to tailor the training routine to the capacity and speed of adaptation of the subject. It should be remembered that the optimal is always what best meets the goals and necessities of the practitioner.

CHAPTER 2
Muscle hypertrophy

Muscle hypertrophy is defined as an increase in the cross-sectional area of the muscle resulting from the repeated exposure of the muscle to a stressor. In the case of training, the stressor is muscle contraction and the acute and chronic responses associated with it.

Within this context, hypertrophy training explores the mechanical tension and metabolic stress (see the following pages), which are perceived by the body as threats to the state of dynamic equilibrium and to the integrity of cells. Thus, physiological responses are organized in order to promote structural adaptations that permit the body to withstand new stressors with less suffering. In the specific case of muscle hypertrophy, these adaptations consist of an increase in the cross-sectional area of skeletal muscle.

This increase is the result of two factors (Guedes Jr. et al., 2008):

- Muscle fiber hypertrophy characterized by an increase in the cross-sectional area of muscle fibers due to an increase in the size and number of myofibrils.
- Muscle fiber hyperplasia characterized by an increase in the number of muscle fibers.

Among these two phenomena, fiber hypertrophy seems to be the main factor responsible for the increase in muscle size. There is still no strong evidence that hyperplasia occurs under normal conditions in humans (Teixeira and Guedes Jr., 2009) and, even if it does, hyperplasia does not account for more than 5% of the total increase in muscle mass (Fleck and Kraemer, 2006).

Mechanical tension

Prior to the understanding of the different types of stress, it should be emphasized that mechanical tension and metabolic stress occur simultaneously, i.e., it is impossible for an exercise or a training technique to explore exclusively one type of stress. However, the combination of acute training variables permits emphasis on mechanical tension or metabolic stress, with both types having a similar potential to promote muscle hypertrophy (Mitchell et al., 2012; Schoenfeld, 2013).

One mechanism whereby resistance exercise stimulates hypertrophy is mechanical tension. As the name implies, it is related to the elevated level of tension imposed on skeletal muscle. To explore mechanical tension, the conventional approach is training with heavy external loads. The characteristics of this training are summarized below:

- Heavy loads: generally higher than 60% of one repetition maximum (1RM).
- Few repetitions: usually less than 8-10RM.
- Long intervals: usually 1-3 minutes.
- Emphasis on eccentric actions.

The stimulation of myofibrillar protein synthesis by mechanical tension is mainly the result of two factors (Schoenfeld, 2010):

- Mechanotransduction: transformation of mechanical energy (muscle contraction) into chemical signals that trigger the Akt/mTOR pathways (myofibrillar protein synthesis).
- Microtraumas (sarcolemma, sarcomere) caused by muscle contraction with an overload (especially eccentric), inducing inflammation and the proliferation and migration of satellite cells.

Mechanical tension has been most frequently reported in classical recommendations of training for muscle hypertrophy, which propose the use of heavy loads, between 60 and 100% of 1RM (ACSM, 2009).

Metabolic stress

Another way of stimulating muscle hypertrophy through resistance training is metabolic stress. In this type of training, the loads used are generally lighter, the time under tension is increased, and the intervals between sets are reduced as summarized below:

- Light/moderate loads: generally less than 60% of 1RM.
- Many repetitions: usually more than 15RM.
- Short intervals: usually less than 1 minute.
- Emphasis on concentric and isometric actions.

In a common hypertrophy resistance program, the duration of the sets ranges from 20 to 40 seconds. The main metabolic route mobilized for the execution of muscle contractions of this duration is the lactic anaerobic pathway (anaerobic glycolysis). The utilization of glucose as an energy source through anaerobic metabolism contributes to increase metabolites in the intracellular medium (lactate, H^+). If the intervals were not sufficient to remove these metabolites, their intracellular levels tend to increase during each set, which could be an important stimulus to trigger protein synthesis. Additionally, the accumulation of metabolites can cause cell swelling, a factor that also contributes to increase the rate of protein synthesis.

Furthermore, prolonged periods of muscle contractions associated with short intervals between sets lead to an environment of ischemia and hypoxia in the muscle (reduced supply of blood and oxygen), increasing the production of reactive oxygen species and the secretion of hormones involved in the process of muscle hypertrophy.

In summary, metabolic stress is related to the depletion of energy substrates, intracellular accumulation of metabolites, cell swelling, ischemia, hypoxia, and increased production of reactive oxygen species (Schoenfeld, 2010).

Despite the common belief to use heavy loads for muscle hypertrophy, recent studies have shown that the use of light loads (e.g., 30% of 1RM), as long as they are mobilized until voluntary fatigue, can elicit acute and chronic responses similar to those seen in traditional hypertrophy training in terms of myofibrillar protein synthesis signaling and the increase in muscle cross-sectional area. These responses are observed in both beginners (Burd et al., 2012; Loenneke, 2012; Schoenfeld, 2013) and well-trained subjects (Schoenfeld et al., 2015).

Ogborn and Schoenfeld (2014) add that, although smaller, type I muscle fibers exhibit a growth potential (hypertrophy). However, in the tension training model (emphasis on heavy loads), although all fibers are recruited, only type II fibers are maximally stimulated when concentric failure is achieved. The authors argue that, since type I fibers are more resistant to fatigue, they would be able to prolong the effort. However, with the "failure" of type II fibers, the capacity of lifting heavy loads is compromised and the set is interrupted. Consequently, type I fibers are not maximally stimulated. Hence, training until concentric failure with light loads in given periods may promote greater stimuli to this type of fiber and may consequently enhance the contribution of these fibers to increase the cross-sectional area of the muscle as a whole.

CHAPTER 3
Advanced training techniques

A training technique is defined as a combination of acute training variables (exercises, order, sets, repetitions, intervals between sets, speed of execution, muscle actions) that provide different physiological and motivational stimuli. Since training variation is a real need, these techniques have been given importance in weight training gyms, especially among experienced practitioners.

As stated in the introduction of this book, most training techniques were developed by practitioners and coaches of past decades, particularly those involved in bodybuilding. The idea has always been focused on maximizing muscle hypertrophy.

At that time, as the understanding of exercise physiology was at the beginning, the basis for development of training techniques was empiricism. Failed attempts were modified until the results were satisfactory. Thus, practical experience and the results observed by those who developed and practiced the techniques served as support for disseminating them throughout the world.

Today, there is growing interest of the scientific community in investigating these different weight training techniques in order to provide, in addition to practical support, the scientific basis for a better understanding, targeting and use of these techniques for hypertrophy. Although recent, this interest has already contributed to some important elucidations.

In this respect, the following pages will explore technical concepts and scientific evidence on advanced weight training techniques. It should be noted that this material is not intended to put an end to all doubts about these techniques, but rather to show what is available in terms of quality information and to encourage future investigations.

The criterion for inclusion of the techniques in this book was the finding of scientific evidence on muscle hypertrophy and related aspects. Thus, many popular techniques are not cited since no studies of these methods and their effects on hypertrophy were found. However, this does not mean that the techniques are not effective for hypertrophy.

The techniques reported will be divided according to the main characteristic related to the type of stress emphasized. Thus, the divisions include techniques that emphasize mechanical tension, techniques that emphasize metabolic stress, mixed techniques (exploring the two types of stress), and undefined techniques (which can be performed by emphasizing either type of stress depending on which variables are manipulated). Importantly, mechanical tension and metabolic stress are intermingled in the process of hypertrophy stimulation. The division proposed in this book is based on emphasis and not on the exclusiveness of stress in order to permit better definition of the characteristics of the training sessions, enabling more conscious and consistent variations. This division is not rigid and it is therefore possible to explore the techniques in ways different from those mentioned in this book.

Techniques that emphasize mechanical tension

Negative repetitions

- Objectives: To emphasize the eccentric phase in order to increase tension levels and consequently the incidence of microtraumas and mechanotransduction.
- Execution: The technique is based on the use of loads greater than 1RM (supramaximal) in order to explore the higher tension levels observed in eccentric actions. The loads usually vary from 105 to 125% of 1RM. For load lifting, the training partner assists in the lift during the concentric phase and the practitioner performs the eccentric phase alone (generally at slow/controlled velocities). The exercise should be performed until eccentric failure (the inability to control the velocity during the eccentric phase).
- Scientific evidence: According to Schoenfeld (2011), most studies claim that eccentric training provides greater hypertrophic gains than concentric or isometric training. The author also states that

eccentric training is associated with a faster response of protein synthesis, higher expression of IGF-1, and more pronounced levels of p70s6k. The likely explanation is the higher incidence of microtraumas and induction of the inflammatory process. Keogh et al. (1999) compared the efficacy of some techniques in terms of acute variables related to strength and hypertrophy and concluded that negative training can be interesting for hypertrophy because it is associated with a longer time under tension than other techniques. Despite these results, few studies have investigated the effects of eccentric training with supramaximal loads using traditional equipment (e.g., free weights), especially in a chronic context. In an attempt to synthesize the results of previous studies, Roig et al. (2009) conducted a systematic review with meta-analysis that compared the efficacy of concentric and eccentric training in increasing muscle mass. Although a small number of the original studies have used protocols similar to that suggested in this book (supramaximal loads), the results suggest that eccentric training with heavy loads is more effective than concentric training in promoting an increase in arm girth and muscle cross-sectional area.

- Author's comments: Because heavy loads are lifted, the technique should be used exclusively by advanced subjects since the stress placed on the joints is extremely high. Considering the high levels of tension observed, the number of repetitions and sets (volume) is generally low, as is the weekly frequency of training for each muscle group. Emphasis on the eccentric phase tends to cause delayed-onset muscle soreness, suggesting its exclusive application to subjects who tolerate this condition.

Forced repetitions

- Objectives: To increase the time under tension in response to the lifting of heavy loads assisted by a training partner.
- Execution: The exercise set is performed until concentric failure; then two or three additional repetitions are performed with the help of a training partner during the concentric phase. The eccentric phase is performed without assistance. A possible variation of the technique consists of the execution of forced repetitions (with assistance) until eccentric failure. Heavy loads are generally used, characterizing the emphasis on mechanical tension.
- Scientific evidence: Frois and Gentil (2011) conducted a literature review including five original articles directly related to the technique. The authors concluded that this technique is effective in promoting an increase in the secretion of growth hormone (GH)

and testosterone, in addition to imposing greater stress on the muscle than traditional methods, causing more microtraumas. However, further longitudinal studies on this technique are needed.

- Author's comments: The execution of repetitions after concentric failure tends to compromise the movement technique. Therefore, this method should be used by subjects who have full control of the exercise techniques. Considering the increased stress imposed on the organism, it is not advisable to perform the technique for prolonged periods.

Rest-pause

- Objectives: To permit an increase in training volume under high-intensity conditions through small recovery intervals within the set.
- Execution: Using heavy loads, repetitions are performed until concentric failure. After failure, the subject rests for 5 to 15 seconds and resumes the set, again performing repetitions until concentric failure. The rest-pause procedure can be repeated two or three times or until the subject is no longer able to perform the repetitions. Example:

Set	Repetitions/intervals
1st	6-8RM
	10" interval
	Repetitions until failure
	10" interval
	Repetitions until failure
Interval	
2nd	...

- Scientific evidence: Most studies on the rest-pause procedure have used the technique in a manner different from that proposed in this book, adopting intervals between repetitions, which does not seem to be interesting for muscle hypertrophy (Giessing et al., 2014). Few studies have investigated the effects of this technique as proposed here. Marshall et al. (2012) compared the effects of three different techniques involving squat exercise on the activation of the thigh and hip muscles and determined the level of post-exercise fatigue. The techniques were: traditional protocol with long intervals (5 sets of 4 repetitions with 3-minute rest intervals between sets), traditional protocol with short intervals (5 sets of 4 repetitions with 20-second rest intervals between sets), and rest-pause training (initial set performed until failure, followed by a 20-second interval and new execution to failure, repeated until a total volume of 20 repetitions is reached). The load used in the three techniques was 80% of 1RM. The rest-pause procedure elicited the best levels of muscle activation without inducing greater post-exercise fatigue. In this respect, one may speculate that the technique is interesting for hypertrophy due to the increased muscle activation. Longitudinal studies are necessary to confirm this hypothesis.

- Author's comments: Continuation of the repetitions after concentric failure tends to compromise the movement technique. Thus, this method should be aimed at subjects who have full control of the exercise techniques. High tension levels maintained for longer periods than normal tend to excessively raise blood pressure and, in view of the interruption of the stimulus, a "rebound" answer of the organism may occur, drastically reducing pressure levels and causing dizziness after the set.

Techniques that emphasize metabolic stress

Partial vascular occlusion (Kaatsu training)

- Objectives: To increase the metabolic stress and level of muscle activation in training programs with light loads by performing exercises under blood flow restriction.

- Execution: The blood flow is restricted (complete occlusion of venous flow and partial occlusion of arterial flow) by placing an inflatable cuff connected to a manometer on the proximal portion of the extremity to be moved during exercise (arms: close to the axilla; thighs: close to the inguinal ligament). The cuff should be inflated until a pressure of 60-80% of the total occlusion pressure or a value of 50 to 200 mmHg is reached. The exercise is performed in this condition using light loads (generally 20 to 50% of 1RM) and maintaining the pressure during the exercise performed until concentric failure. The pressure is maintained throughout the sets of the same exercise (2 to 4 sets) and is removed when the exercise is changed. Short rest intervals are adopted between sets of the same exercise (30-60 seconds) and long intervals between exercises (approximately 5 minutes).

- Scientific evidence: Kaatsu training has been one of the most investigated techniques in recent years and the results demonstrate that its use is effective and safe. In order to synthesize the results of previously conducted research, Pope et al. (2013) published a short review on the technique, summarizing its physiological, morphological and functional effects. The authors concluded that training with light loads associated with vascular occlusion provides

33

adaptations similar to those seen in training with heavy loads (increases in strength and muscle mass), and that this protocol would be interesting for individuals who do not wish to lift heavy loads because of physical restriction or momentary option. An interesting fact is that the adaptations are observed not only in muscles proximal to the occlusion, but also in distal muscles. Scott et al. (2015) added that the training results of healthy subjects can be maximized if the technique were combined/alternated with traditional training using heavy loads. The use of alternative materials for vascular occlusion (e.g., knee wraps) has been investigated and, so far, as long as the pressure is controlled, the technique seems to be equally safe and effective (Wilson et al., 2013; Lowery et al., 2014). In the case of knee wraps, Wilson et al. (2013) suggested the adoption of a scale of subjective pressure perception ranging from 0 to 10. A score of 7 on this scale seems to be ideal for training (pressure sensation without pain).

- Author's comments: Blood flow restriction increases the accumulation of metabolites in the muscle, enhancing the acute sensation of pain and burning. The method should therefore be applied only to subjects who tolerate this condition. In view of the light loads and reduced volume compared to the situation without vascular occlusion, the overload on the joints and noncontractile structures is attenuated. The occlusion pressure should be adjusted during each set. It is suggested to read in full the articles cited above before practical application of the technique, regardless of the equipment used.

Isodynamic (adapted vascular occlusion)

- Objectives: To increase the metabolic stress in training programs with light loads through maximum isometric contraction prior to the dynamic set.
- Execution: A maximum isometric voluntary contraction is sustained for 15 to 20 seconds at the point of maximum shortening (or near it) of the muscle to be trained (the isometric exercise does not necessarily be performed in the same exercise that will be subsequently executed). Immediately after isometric exercise, the dynamic execution of the movement is initiated (for the same muscle group) until concentric failure using light to moderate loads. Example: maximal isometric contraction of the chest on the pec deck for 20 seconds, followed by a dynamic bench press set.
- Scientific evidence: This technique has been proposed as an alternative to Kaatsu training since it is speculated that previous sustained isometric exercise generates a state of ischemia and hypoxia for the

execution of subsequent repetitions in this condition. However, original studies on this technique are scarce in the literature. Gentil et al. (2006a) compared the effects of different training techniques on acute blood lactate responses and load characteristics. The time under tension was greater for isodynamic training when compared to the traditional methods (10RM and 6RM) and forced repetitions, in addition to providing higher total work than the traditional methods. All techniques significantly increased blood lactate levels compared to rest, without a statistical difference between techniques. Despite the lack of a significant difference, it should be noted that absolute lactate levels were higher for the isodynamic technique and functional isometrics compared to the other methods. In another study, Gentil et al. (2006b) confirmed a higher magnitude of metabolic stress for the isodynamic technique and functional isometrics, with the observation of significantly higher blood lactate levels compared to the 10RM and super-slow techniques. Further studies evaluating the chronic effects of the technique are necessary.

- Author's comments: Previous isometric exercise generates a state of ischemia and hypoxia due to blood vessel collapse, increasing the sensation of pain and burning prior to the execution of a set. This may compromise the dynamic movement technique due to fatigue. This method should therefore be aimed at subjects who have full control of the exercise techniques. Continuous respiration should be encouraged during the isometric exercise to attenuate the blood pressure responses.

Functional isometrics

- Objectives: To increase the metabolic stress in training programs with light loads through isometric contractions amidst dynamic repetitions of the set.
- Execution: Using light to moderate loads, the proposed set is executed by performing isometric actions lasting 2 to 3 seconds at the end of each concentric phase or at the point of maximum tension.
- Scientific evidence: Gentil et al. (2006a,b) compared the effects of different training techniques on acute blood lactate responses and load characteristics. Functional isometrics provided results similar to those of isodynamic training (discussed above) and might be an option for substitution/variation. Keogh et al. (1999) observed that functional isometrics resulted in higher acute concentric force production and similar levels of muscle activation, eccentric force and time under tension compared to the traditional method in bench press exercise. The authors speculate that the technique could be more effective than the traditional

method for muscle hypertroph, but recognize the need for longitudinal studies to confirm this hypothesis.

- Author's comments: The use of this technique should be avoided in exercises that present a moment of rest at the end of the concentric phase (e.g., bench press, squat) since isometrics would be unproductive at this point. In the case of these exercises, one option is to perform isometric exercise at the point of greatest resistance moment arm (point of maximum tension), a technique known by some as functional isometrics.

Supersets

- Objectives: To increase the time of the stimulus through sequential exercises for the same muscle group without intervals between exercises, and to stimulate different muscle fibers in the same set through different exercises for the same muscle group.
- Execution: Two or more exercises for the same muscle group are performed sequentially without intervals between them. Example: a set of squat exercises, followed without interval by a set of leg press exercises. The supersets can be classified as bi-set (two sequential exercises), tri-set (three exercises), or giant set (four or more exercises). Example:

Superset	1st set		2nd set
Bi-set	SQ + LP	Interval	...
Tri-set	SP + FR + LR		...
Giant set	BP + IBP + DBP + CF		...

SQ: squat; LP: leg press; SP: shoulder press; FR: front raise; LR: lateral raise; BP: bench press; IBP: inclined bench press; DBP: declined bench press; CF: chest fly.

- Scientific evidence: Ceola and Tumerelo (2008) investigated the effects of supersets on muscle hypertrophy evaluated by girth measurements after 4 and 8 weeks of training, comparing the results with the traditional method. The results showed more pronounced increases in girths in the first 4 weeks of giant set training; however, after 8 weeks, superior results were obtained with the traditional method. The authors concluded that, for rapid increases in body girths, supersets seem to be more effective, but the technique loses efficiency compared to the traditional method if the training program exceeds 4 weeks. Uchida et al. (2006) compared the effects of tri-set and multiple-set (traditional) techniques on structural and hormonal alterations after 8 weeks of training. The authors found no significant changes in the structural variables, but observed that the tri-set technique imposed more stress on the organism, acutely and chronically increasing serum cortisol levels and reducing the testosterone/cortisol ratio. In contrast, the traditional method led to a more favorable hormone environment for anabolism.

- Author's comments: Because of the sequential execution of the exercises without rest intervals, the level of stress seems to increase from the bi-set to the giant set. It would be interesting to adopt a progression scheme in this order if the superset technique were to be introduced in the program of weight lifting practitioners. In view of the high level of stress imposed by the method, it should be applied for short periods of time (shock microcycles), followed by recovery (restorative microcycles), considering the results of the studies cited above.

Decreasing rest intervals

- Objectives: To increase the metabolic stress while decreasing external training loads at the cost of reducing the inter-set interval during the weeks of training.
- Execution: A fixed RM zone is established and kept over a few weeks (e.g., 8 to 10RM; 8 weeks). Exercise is initiated with heavy loads and long inter-set intervals (e.g., 2 minutes). The inter-set interval is then reduced by 15 seconds per week until reaching the limit of 30 seconds. If necessary, the external load can be

reduced for adaptation to the initially proposed RM zone. Example:

Week	1st	2nd	3rd	4th	5th
Sets	4	4	4	4	4
RM	8-10	8-10	8-10	8-10	8-10
Intervals	1'30"	1'15"	1'	45"	30"

- Scientific evidence: Souza Junior et al. (2010) compared the effects of two training techniques on maximal strength in bench press and squat exercises and on arm and thigh cross-sectional area in 20 recreationally trained men. The training protocol had a duration of 8 weeks and the subjects were divided into two groups according to the interval between sets: four sets of 8-10RM with 2-minute rest intervals between sets (G1); four sets of 8-10RM with 2-minute rest intervals between sets that were decreased by 15 seconds per week after the third week (G2). To maintain the training volume within the proposed zone, G2 significantly decreased the loads lifted after the 4th week. The results showed that, even with the significant decrease in the weight lifted, both groups increased strength and cross-sectional area, without a significant difference between groups. More recently, another study using a similar training technique, but creatine supplementation in the two groups, reported the same results (Souza Junior et al., 2011).

- Author's comments: The reduction in external training load is one of the major difficulties encountered by weight training professionals since the "vanity" component is very strong in this environment. This technique is very productive in this respect since shortening the intervals between sets forces a load reduction without compromising the results. This could be an interesting strategy for practitioners who have long been exploring heavy sets and who desire to gradually modify their training in order to emphasize metabolic stress.

Mixed techniques

Drop sets

- Objectives: To increase the time under tension and total work, permitting the execution of more repetitions because of the load reduction amidst the set; to explore mechanical tension at the beginning of the set and metabolic stress at the end of the set.
- Execution: The exercise is initiated with heavy loads and repetitions are performed until concentric failure. After failure, the load is reduced (by about 10 to 20%) and the exercise is resumed without interval and again

performed until concentric failure. The procedure of external load reduction can be repeated two or three times or until the training objectives are achieved. Example:

Set	Repetitions	Load
1st	5-7RM	80 kg
	Until failure	65 kg
	Until failure	50 kg
Interval		
2nd	Repeat	Repeat
...	...	...

- Scientific evidence: Keogh et al. (1999) observed that, in the drop set, the load reduction after fatigue permits to maintain a good level of muscle activation for prolonged periods, a fact that makes the technique interesting for enhancing muscle hypertrophy. Gentil et al. (2006a) compared the effects of different training techniques on acute blood lactate responses and load characteristics. The results revealed that the drop set produced a longer time under tension and greater total overload (total volume of load lifted) than the other techniques studied. The drop set is therefore an effective technique in promoting high levels of muscle stress and, supposedly, subsequent hypertrophy. Goto et al. (2003) showed that the drop set (in that study:

execution of a set of low-intensity resistance exercise immediately after a set of high-intensity exercise) resulted in a higher increase in GH concentrations than the exclusive execution of a set of high-intensity exercise. Subsequently, the same group of researchers (Goto et al., 2004) found that the addition of a drop in the final set of a traditional training model contributed to an expressive increase in muscle cross-sectional area, which was not observed for the traditional model. Another study (Eichmann and Giessing, 2013) compared the effects of drop sets and traditional training on the gains in strength and muscle mass of trained subjects after 10 weeks of intervention. For this purpose, the subjects were divided into three groups: one drop set of each exercise until concentric failure; three traditional sets of each exercise until concentric failure, and control. The results showed an increase in strength and muscle mass in the two training groups; however, the drop set provided better responses despite the smaller number of sets. It should be noted that the last study was published in abstract form, a fact impairing more detailed analysis of the techniques used. According to Ogborn and Schoenfeld (2014), a likely explanation is that the load reduction after fatigue permits to prolong the stimuli to type I fibers, increasing their contribution to muscle hypertrophy.

- Author's comments: It is advisable to perform the exercise in equipment with loading systems that use columns or blocks since this facilitates and speeds up the load reduction. Because of the high stress imposed by the technique (long time under tension, high total work), drop sets should not be performed for prolonged periods of time to avoid overtraining.

Ascending pyramid

- Objectives: To prepare the musculature to withstand an increasing intensity during the training session by progressively increasing the load with each set; to explore metabolic stress at the beginning of exercise and mechanical tension at the end of exercise.
- Execution: The first set of exercise is performed with light/moderate loads and an interval is allowed between sets. The load is increased progressively with each subsequent set and the number of repetitions is reduced. No rule exists for the increase in load, but it is generally increased by 10 to 20%. Example:

Set	Repetitions	Load	Interval
1st	11-13RM	80 kg	1'
2nd	9-11RM	90 kg	1'30"
3rd	7-9RM	100 kg	2'
4th	5-7RM	110 kg	2'30"

- Scientific evidence: Since the basic premise to explore mechanical tension is the amount of load lifted, the efficiency of this technique can be questioned since in the last sets, in which the objective is to increase the load, previous fatigue compromises the ability of weight lifting and consequently reduces the utilization of mechanical tension. However, De Salles et al. (2008a) observed no significant differences in the number of repetitions between ascending and descending pyramid training with the same load configurations. In that study, the loads used were 70, 80 and 90% of 1RM in leg extension exercise. The subjects performed the exercise in two different orders (from the lighter to the heavier one and vice-versa), with fixed rest intervals of 3 minutes between sets. In another study, Da Silva et al. (2010) found similar levels of creatine kinase after ascending and descending pyramid training, suggesting that the two techniques are equally effective in promoting microtraumas and the subsequent inflammatory process, an important inducer of muscle hypertrophy.

It should be noted that the ascending pyramid model used in the study of Da Silva et al. (2010) was originally proposed by Thomas DeLorme. In this model, only the load was increased, while the number of repetitions was maintained constant at 10 (the first two sets were performed in a submaximal manner and only the last set was performed until failure). The authors concluded that the choice of one technique or the other should be at the discretion of the coach since both seem to elicit similar responses. Charro et al. (2010) compared the acute metabolic, hormonal and perceptual responses of recreationally trained subjects between ascending pyramid training and multiple sets. The techniques were matched for the total volume of load lifted. The results showed no significant differences between techniques. The same group of researchers (Charro et al., 2012) conducted a similar study to compare the effects on acute markers of muscle damage. Similarly, the results revealed no difference between techniques. Gentil (2011) alerted that, even in view of the load increase, the repetitions should be kept within the zone recommended for muscle hypertrophy in order to avoid deconfiguration of the training objective.

- Author's comments: In the condition of previous fatigue, the load increase may compromise the movement technique, increasing the risk of injury. The method should therefore be aimed at subjects who have extensive control of the techniques. Ascending pyramid training may be an interesting strategy for practitioners who have long been exploring sets with many repetitions and who desire to gradually modify their training in order to emphasize mechanical tension.

Descending pyramid

- Objectives: To take advantage of the initial rest state to lift heavy weights, reducing the load with progression of the set appropriate for the situation of fatigue; to explore mechanical tension at the beginning of exercise and metabolic stress at the end of exercise.
- Execution: The first set of exercise is performed with heavy loads and an interval is allowed between sets. The load is reduced progressively with each subsequent set and the number of repetitions is increased. No rule exists for the reduction in load, but it is generally reduced by 10 to 20%. Example:

Set	Repetitions	Load	Interval
1st	5-7RM	110 kg	2'30"
2nd	7-9RM	100 kg	2'
3rd	9-11RM	90 kg	1'30"
4th	11-13RM	80 kg	1'

- Scientific evidence: Since the basic premise to explore mechanical tension is the amount of the load lifted, Gentil (2011) suggests the performance of descending pyramid training to be better than that of the ascending pyramid since heavier loads are lifted in the initial sets. With the onset of fatigue, the loads are reduced and metabolic stress starts to be emphasized. However, as mentioned for the previous technique, De Salles et al. (2008a) did not observe significant differences in the number of repetitions between ascending and descending pyramid training using the same load configurations and fixed rest intervals of 3 minutes between sets, suggesting the benefits of the different types of stress to be similar for the two techniques. In another study, Da Silva et al. (2010) found similar levels of creatine kinase after ascending and descending pyramid training, suggesting that the two methods are equally effective in promoting microtraumas and the subsequent inflammatory process, an important inducer of muscle hypertrophy. It should be noted that in the originally proposed

(Oxford) descending pyramid model used in the study of Da Silva et al. (2010), only the load was reduced, while the number of repetitions was maintained constant at 10 (only the first set was performed until failure, while the last two sets were submaximal). The authors concluded that the choice of one technique or the other should be at the discretion of the coach since both seem to elicit similar responses. Longitudinal studies involving the pyramid techniques are needed.

• Author's comments: Descending pyramid training permits the lift of heavy weights in a situation of rest, facilitating the movement technique, and is therefore interesting for subjects who are starting to use advanced training techniques. The method could be interesting for practitioners who have long been exploring heavy sets and who desire to gradually modify their training in order to emphasize metabolic stress. An interesting strategy for stimulus definition is the use of the technique during the session (more load in the first exercises and less load in the last exercises) rather than per exercise.

Pre-exhaustion

• Objectives: As in multi-joint exercises, several muscle groups are recruited and the exercise is interrupted because of fatigue of the muscles that are not considered major in the exercise. Thus, the objective is to generate fatigue in the target muscle (metabolic stress) prior to execution of the main exercise so that the muscle is more requested in the last exercise (mechanical tension).

- Execution: A single-joint exercise is performed prior to a multi-joint exercise involving the same muscle group. Example: chest fly before bench press to induce fatigue of the pectoralis muscle prior to the main exercise; knee extension before squat to induce fatigue of the quadriceps muscle prior to the main exercise.

- Scientific evidence: The neuromuscular recruitment pattern is altered in the presence of fatigue, favoring the activation of muscles that are not fatigued (Behm and St-Pierre, 1997). This idea was considered by Augustsson et al. (2003) who analyzed the level of activation of the rectus femoris, vastus lateralis, and gluteus maximus muscles in two conditions of a leg press exercise: with pre-exhaustion (knee extension followed by leg press exercise) and without pre-exhaustion. The authors observed lower activation of the quadriceps muscles during the leg press exercise when it was preceded by knee extension, while no significant difference was found for the gluteus maximus. Another study (Gentil et al., 2007) investigated the effects of pre-exhaustion on the pattern of activation of the pectoralis, anterior deltoid and triceps brachii muscles in two different exercise orders: pec deck + bench press (pre-exhaustion) versus bench press + pec deck (post-exhaustion). Despite the lack of a significant change, in the pre-exhaustion condition activation of the pectoralis muscle exhibited a delta of -5.44% in the bench press, while activation of the triceps brachii increased significantly by 33.67%. No significant differences were found for deltoid EMG. Simão et al. (2012) concluded in a review on the effects of exercise order that pre-exhaustion is not an effective technique when the objective is to increase the neuromuscular recruitment of large muscle groups in the "main" exercises. However, De Salles et al. (2008b) observed that in the pre-exhaustion condition the total number of repetitions for the lower extremities was higher than in the reverse order, a fact that could increase stress and assist in hypertrophic responses. More recently, Fisher et al. (2014) compared the effects of three different interventions on the strength and lean mass of trained subjects over a period of 12 weeks: pre-exhaustion without a rest interval between exercises, pre-exhaustion with a rest interval between exercises, and post-exhaustion. The results showed that all techniques were effective in increasing strength levels, without a significant difference between techniques.

None of the methods promoted significant changes in lean mass.

- Author's comments: Although pre-exhaustion exercise does not exhibit effectiveness in terms of the activation of large muscle groups, this technique seems to be effective in increasing the recruitment of small muscle groups (at least in the bench press) and is an interesting strategy when the desire is to emphasize the work of these muscle in basic (multi-joint) exercises.

Post-exhaustion (priority)

- Objectives: As in multi-joint exercises, several muscle groups are activated and the interruption of exercise is the result of fatigue of the muscles that are not considered major in the exercise. Thus, the objective is to continue stimulating the target muscle (metabolic stress) through a single-joint exercise after interruption (due to fatigue) of the multi-joint exercise (mechanical tension).
- Execution: A single-joint exercise is performed after a multi-joint exercise involving the same muscle group. Example: chest fly immediately after bench press to continue stimulating the pectoralis muscle; knee extension immediately after squat to continue stimulating the quadriceps muscle.

- Scientific evidence: Gentil et al. (2007) observed that a prior bench press exercise (before pec deck) permitted the execution of more repetitions of the exercise compared to the reverse order. Considering the bench press to be one of the main exercises, the post-exhaustion technique becomes more interesting than the reverse. Furthermore, the authors observed that activation of the pectoralis muscle tended to be higher in the post-exhaustion (priority) exercise compared to the pre-exhaustion condition. However, in the study conducted by Fisher et al. (2014) comparing the effects of three different interventions on the strength and lean mass of trained subjects (pre-exhaustion without a rest interval between exercises, pre-exhaustion with a rest interval between exercises, and post-exhaustion) over a period of 12 weeks, all techniques were effective in increasing strength levels, with no significant difference between techniques. Regarding lean mass, none of the methods promoted significant changes.

- Author's comments: The lifting of heavy loads in multi-joint exercise is maximized since the exercise is performed in a situation of rest. It is therefore possible to define the stimuli in the session, progressing from mechanical tension (multi-joint) to metabolic stress (single-joint). Since it facilitates the movement technique (a heavier load at the beginning through multi-joint exercise, a lighter load at the end through single-joint exercise), post-exhaustion training may be an interesting option for subjects who are starting to use advanced training techniques.

Undefined techniques

Agonist-antagonist

- Objectives: To optimize the training duration by taking advantage of the inter-set intervals to work antagonist muscles; to stimulate the redirection of blood flow to a specific body region in order to facilitate the supply of oxygen and nutrients to potentiate performance and outcomes; to take advantage of the reduced coactivation to maximize muscle tension.
- Execution: Two exercises for antagonist muscles are performed in a paired manner, taking advantage of the rest interval of one to execute the other. The exercises can be performed with or without a short interval between them. Example:

Muscle	1st set	Interval	2nd set	Interval	...
Biceps	BC		BC		...

Triceps	Interval	TP	Interval	TP	...
Muscle		1st set		2nd set	...

BC: biceps curl; TP: triceps pushdown.

- Scientific evidence: Nobre et al. (2010) observed improvement of acute knee extension performance when the exercise was preceded by a set of knee flexion. The authors investigated the acute performance in a 10RM knee extension test with or without previous 10RM knee flexion exercise. In the paired condition, the average performance increased to 13 repetitions, suggesting that previous fatigue of the antagonist muscle can potentiate agonist performance. Similar results have been reported by Machado et al. (2007) who investigated elbow flexion performance with a load of 80% of 1RM using two different warm-up protocols: two sets of 12 repetitions of elbow flexion with 60% of 1RM and a 1-minute interval between sets; two sets of 12 repetitions of elbow extension with 60% of 1RM and a 1-minute interval between sets. The maximum repetition test using 80% of 1RM exhibited the best performance when it was preceded by warm-up of the antagonist muscle (10.86 *vs* 7.66 repetitions). Paz et al. (2014)

also observed an increase in the total training volume (total repetitions) in the agonist-antagonist scheme compared to the traditional method in bench press and wide grip row exercises, in addition to increased activation of the muscles involved in the second exercise. This increase in the number of repetitions for the same load configurations may be interesting to increase muscle stress and, consequently, hypertrophic responses (Schoenfeld, 2011). Robbins et al. (2010) concluded that agonist-antagonist training increases the training density, permitting the execution of a larger number of repetitions in less time without altering exercise intensity. The time-efficient characteristic may be suitable for subjects who have less time available for training. In addition, the higher density may contribute to increase muscle stress levels, which is important for hypertrophy stimulation, but longitudinal studies are necessary. It should be noted that the effects of this technique are more evident in the subsequently performed exercises/muscles (after the antagonist exercise). With respect to rest intervals between exercises in the paired set, Maia et al. (2014) observed better acute responses in terms of the number of repetitions performed and electromyographic signal when no rest or short rest intervals (e.g., 30 seconds and 1 minute) were adopted.

- Author's comments: The technique is undefined because it can be used to emphasize either mechanical tension or metabolic stress according to the configuration adopted for manipulation of the training variables. The stress does not necessarily need to be the same for the antagonist muscle and can follow the sequence: tension/tension, metabolic/metabolic, tension/metabolic, and metabolic/tension. The sensation of pumping is enhanced because of the increased redirection of blood flow to the exercised region. The choice of the exercise should consider the planes and axes of movement in order to select truly antagonistic exercises (e.g., bench press and wide grip row; biceps curl and triceps pushdown; wide grip shoulder press and wide grip lateral pulldown).

Agonist- contralateral antagonist

- Objectives: To increase muscle tension as a result of the simultaneous activation of the contralateral antagonists, and to reduce bilateral deficit.
- Execution: Antagonist exercises of the contralateral limbs are performed simultaneously. The movements of the segments involved are exactly the same from a kinematics point of view, but differ in the application of force (kinetics). Example: right elbow flexion with

dumbbell is performed simultaneously to left triceps pushdown, synchronizing concentric and eccentric actions.

- Scientific evidence: Weineck (2003), citing Adam and Werchoshanskij (1974), states that in elbow flexion exercise the tension of left arm flexion – and also the training stimulus – is enhanced if the right arm extensor muscles were tensioned simultaneously. This statement is supported by Ohtsuki (1983) who identified that the bilateral deficit is reduced when the contralateral antagonist is activated. This author observed an enhanced electromyographic signal in the left triceps in response to voluntary contraction of the right biceps brachii compared to rest, even when the former is relaxed. This is due to the phenomenon of coactivation (simultaneous activation of agonists and antagonists) and cross-innervation. Thus, if the contralateral antagonists were activated simultaneously, muscle tension is increased due to contralateral antagonist coactivation. This feature can increase stress and the resulting hypertrophic stimuli. However, longitudinal studies are needed to verify the effects of this technique on muscle mass.

- Author's comments: The technique is undefined because it can be used to emphasize mechanical tension or metabolic stress according to the configuration adopted for manipulation of the training variables. The simultaneous performance of the contralateral antagonists increases the requirements for the neuromuscular system, thus increasing complexity. The method should therefore be applied to experienced subjects to avoid compromising the movement technique. Practical research performed during courses (unpublished data) has shown that the technique permits an increase in volume (repetitions) for the same load when compared to unilateral execution of a given exercise. The application of force to the limbs in opposite directions generates perturbations to the center of gravity, which could be interesting to potentiate the action on core muscles while exercising other body segments.

Circuit

- Objectives: To increase energy expenditure and participation of the cardiorespiratory component, and to optimize training session duration through the sequential execution of exercises involving large muscle groups by alternating body segments.
- Execution: Six to 10 primarily multi-joint exercises (stations) are selected. The exercises are sequenced in a way to alternate body segments. The first circuit consists of the sequential execution of one set of each exercise without or with small rest intervals (15 to 30

seconds) between exercises. The circuit is repeated 1, 2 or 3 times, adopting a rest interval of 1 to 3 minutes between circuits. A fixed number of repetitions per exercise (e.g., 15 repetitions) or a predetermined time (e.g., 30 seconds) can be adopted.

- Scientific evidence: The effects related to circuit training have been studied for a long time. Already in the 1970s, Wilmore et al. (1978) showed good results of this technique. In that study, men and women were submitted to a 10-week program of circuit weight training. The circuit consisted of 10 exercises, with 3 circuits per day. The load used ranged from 40-55% of 1RM and the subjects were encouraged to perform as many repetitions as possible in 30 seconds, followed by a 15-second rest interval between exercises. At the end of the intervention, the authors observed a significant increase in lean mass and flexed arm girth and a reduction in skinfold measurements in the experimental groups, in addition to improvement of strength and cardiorespiratory conditioning. No changes were observed in the control group. It should be noted that the mean duration of the training sessions was 22.5 minutes. Recent studies have confirmed the efficacy of the technique. Alcaraz et al. (2011) found that circuit training using loads compatible with 6RM promoted similar muscle mass increases in trained men when compared to traditional training (multiple sets), but optimized training session duration. With respect to energy expenditure during and immediately after the training session, Murphy and Schwarzkopf (1992) found that circuit training promoted better responses than traditional training. In summary, when compared to the traditional method, De Salles and Simão (2014) concluded that circuit training is interesting to promote muscle hypertrophy at a similar magnitude, to maximize the reduction in fat percentage, and to optimize training duration.

- Author's comments: Circuit training is an undefined technique because it can be used to emphasize mechanical tension or metabolic stress according to the configuration adopted for manipulation of the training variables. In view of the possibility to optimize training duration, the technique is an interesting strategy for people who have little time to train. The exercises (stations) should be arranged in such a way to optimize space, i.e., close to one another to facilitate the change between stations. Circuit training should be avoided during peak gym hours since occupation of the equipment by other practitioners and the need for rotation may compromise the dynamics of the method.

FINAL CONSIDERATIONS

Based on the literature reviewed, there is no sufficient scientific evidence to support the superiority of one technique over the other, nor any evidence that discredits any of the techniques described. However, some techniques are distinguished by their proven efficiency, while others require further investigation, especially longitudinal studies. The table below summarizes the techniques whose acute and chronic effects have been investigated.

Investigated effects	Techniques
Acute	Forced repetitions, Rest-pause, Isodynamic, Functional isometrics, Agonist-antagonist, Agonist-contralateral antagonist
Chronic	Negative repetitions, Partial vascular occlusion, Supersets, Decreasing rest intervals, Drop sets, Pre-exhaustion, Post-exhaustion, Pyramid, Circuit

Thus, emphasis should be placed on techniques with already proven chronic effects, especially in medium-/long-term training programs. However, considering the acute effects of some techniques, particularly in terms of direct and indirect markers of stress (tension and metabolic), as well as signaling pathways of myofibrillar protein synthesis, these techniques become interesting options for use in individual phases of a periodization (e.g., shock microcycle).

At this point of the reading, I hope that this information has contributed to a more sensible and conscious use of the different techniques and has served as encouragement to conduct new and more detailed studies on this topic.

REFERENCES

ACSM - AMERICAN COLLEGE OF SPORTS MEDICINE. Position stand: progression models in resistance training for healthy adults. **Medicine and Science in Sports and Exercise**. 41(3): 687-708, 2009.

ALCARAZ, PE; PEREZ-GOMEZ, J; CHAVARRIAS, M; BLAZEVICH, AJ. Similarity in adaptations to high-resistance circuit vs. traditional strength training in resistance trained men. **Journal of Strength and Conditioning Research**. 25: 2519-2527, 2011.

AUGUSTSSON, J; THOMEÉ, R; HORNSTEDT, P; LINDBLOM, J; KARLSSON, J; GRIMBY, G. Effect of pre-exhaustion exercise on lower-extremity muscle activation during a leg press exercise. **Journal of Strength and Conditioning Research**. 17(2): 411-416, 2003.

BEHM, DG; ST-PIERRE, DM. Effects of fatigue duration and muscle type on voluntary and evoked contractile properties. **Journal of Applied Physiology**. 82(5): 1654-1661, 1997.

BURD, NA.; MITCHELL, CJ; CHURCHWARD-VENNE, TA; PHILLIPS, SM. Bigger weights may not beget bigger muscles: evidence from acute muscle protein synthetic responses after resistance exercise. **Applied Physiology, Nutrition, and Metabolism**. 37(3): 551–554, 2012.

CEOLA, MHJ; TUMELERO, S. Grau de hipertrofia muscular em resposta a três métodos de treinamento de força muscular. **Lecturas Educacion Fisica y Deportes**. 13(121), 2008.

CHARRO, MA; AOKI, MS; COUTTS, AJ; ARAUJO, RC; BACURAU, RF. Hormonal, metabolic and perceptual responses to different resistance training systems. **Journal of Sports Medicine and Physical Fitness**. 50: 229-234, 2010.

CHARRO, MA; AOKI, MS; NOSAKA, K; FOSCHINI, D; FIGUEIRA JUNIOR, A; BACURAU, R. Comparison between multiple sets and half-pyramid resistance exercise bouts for muscle damage profiles. **European Journal of Sport Science**. 12(3): 249-254, 2012.

DA SILVA, DP; CURTY, VM; AREAS, JM; SOUZA, SC; HACKNEY, AC; MACHADO, M. Comparison of DeLorme with Oxford resistance training techniques: effects of training on muscle damage markers. **Biology of Sport**. 27(2): 77-81, 2010.

DE SALLES, BF; SILVA, JPM; OLIVEIRA, D; RIBEIRO, FM; SIMÃO, R. Efeito dos métodos pirâmide crescente e pirâmide decrescente no número de repetições do treinamento de força. **Arquivos em Movimento**. 4(1): 23-31, 2008a.

DE SALLES, BF; OLIVEIRA, N; RIBEIRO, FM; SIMÃO, R; NOVAES, JS. Comparação do método pré-exaustão e da ordem inversa em exercícios para membros inferiores. **Revista da Educação Física UEM**. 19(1): 85-92, 2008b.

DE SALLES, BF; SIMÃO, R. Bases científicas dos métodos e sistemas de treinamento de força. **Revista Uniandrade**. 15(2): 127-133, 2014.

EICHMANN, B; GIESSING, J. Effects of ten weeks of either multiple-set training or single-set training on strength and muscle mass. **British Journal of Sports Medicine**. 47: e3, 2013.

FISHER, JP; CARLSON, L.; STEELE, J; SMITH, D. The effects of pre-exhaustion, exercise order, and rest intervals in a full-body resistance training intervention. **Applied Physiology, Nutrition and Metabolism**. 39: 1265-1270, 2014.

FLECK, S. Non-linear periodization for general fitness & athletes. **Journal of Human Kinetics**. 29A: 41-45, 2011.

FLECK, SJ; KRAEMER, WJ. **Fundamentos do treinamento de força muscular**. 3rd ed. Porto Alegre: Artmed, 2006.

GENTIL, P. **Bases científicas do treinamento de hipertrofia.** 4th ed. Rio de Janeiro: Sprint, 2011.

GENTIL, P; OLIVEIRA, E; FONTANA, K; MOLINA, G; OLIVEIRA, RJ; BOTTARO, M. Efeitos agudos de vários métodos de treinamento de força no lactato sanguíneo e características de cargas em homens treinados recreacionalmente. **Revista Brasileira de Medicina do Esporte.** 12(6): 303-307, 2006a.

GENTIL, P; OLIVEIRA, E; BOTTARO, M. Time under tension and blood lactate response during four different resistance training methods. **Journal of Physiological Anthropology.** 25: 339-344, 2006b.

GENTIL, P; OLIVEIRA, E; ROCHA JUNIOR, VA; CARMO, J; BOTTARO, M. Effects of exercise order on upper-body muscle activation and exercise performance. **Journal of Strength and Conditioning Research.** 21(4): 1082-1086, 2007.

GIESSING, J; FISHER, J; STEELE, J; ROTHE, F; RAUBOLD, K; EICHMANN, B. The effects of low volume resistance training with and without advanced techniques in trained participants. **The Journal of Sports Medicine and Physical Fitness.** Epud ahead of print, 2014.

GOTO, K; NAGASAWA, M; YANAGISAWA, O; KIZUKA, T; ISHII, N; TAKAMATSU, K. Muscular adaptations to combinations of high- and low-intensity resistance exercises. **Journal of Strength and Conditioning Research.** 18(4): 730-737, 2004.

GOTO, K; SATO, K; TAKAMATSU, K. A single set of low intensity resistance exercise immediately following high intensity resistance exercise stimulates growth hormone secretion in men. **Journal of Sports Medicine and Physical Fitness.** 43(2): 243-249, 2003.

GUEDES JR., DP; SOUZA JR., TP; ROCHA, AC. **Treinamento personalizado em musculação.** São Paulo: Phorte, 2008.

KEOGH, JWL; WILSON, GJ; WEATHERBY, RP. A cross-sectional comparison of different resistance training techniques in the bench press. **Journal of Strength and Conditioning Research**. 13(3): 247–258, 1999.

LOENNEKE, JP. Skeletal muscle hypertrophy: how important is exercise intensity? **Journal of Trainology**. 2: 28-31, 2012.

LOWERY, RP; JOY, JM; LOENNEKE, JP; DE SOUZA, EO; MACHADO, M; DUDECK, JE; WILSON, JM. Practical blood flow restriction training increases muscle hypertrophy during a periodized resistance training programme. **Clinical Physiology and Functional Imaging**. 34(4): 317-321, 2014.

MACHADO, AF; PANTALEÃO, D; PAIVA, BM; TROYACK, ES. Influência do aquecimento com o músculo agonista e antagonista sobre o número máximo de repetições realizadas. **Coleção Pesquisa em Educação Física**. 6: 331-336, 2007.

MAIA, MF; WILLARDSON, JM; PAZ, GA; MIRANDA, H. Effects of different rest intervals between antagonist paired sets on repetition performance and muscle activation. **Journal of Strength and Conditioning Research**. 28(9): 2529-2535, 2014.

MARSHALL, PWM; ROBBINS, DA; WRIGHTSON, AW; SIEGLER, JC. Acute neuromuscular and fatigue responses to the rest-pause method. Journal of **Science and Medicine in Sport**. 15(2): 153-158, 2012.

MINOZZO, FC; LIRA, CAB; VANCINI, RL; SILVA, AAB; FACHINA, RJFG; GUEDES JR., DP; GOMES, AC; SILVA, AC. Periodização do treinamento de força: uma revisão crítica. **Revista Brasileira de Ciência e Movimento**. 16(1): 89-97, 2008.

MITCHELL, CJ; CHURCHWARD-VENNE, TA; WEST, DWD; BURD, NA; BREEN, L; BAKER, SK; Phillips, SM. Resistance exercise load does not determine training-mediated hypertrophic gains in young men. **Journal of Applied Physiology**. 113(1): 71–77, 2012.

MURPHY, E; SCHWARZKOPF, R. Effects of standard set and circuit weight training on excess post-exercise oxygen consumption. **Journal of Applied Sport Science Research**. 6: 88-91, 1992.

NOBRE, M; FIGUEIREDO, T; SIMÃO, R. Influência do método agonista-antagonista no desempenho do treinamento de força para membros inferiores. **Revista Brasileira de Fisiologia e Prescrição do Exercício**. 4(22): 397-401, 2010.

OGBORN, D; SCHOENFELD, BJ. The role of fiber types in muscle hypertrophy: implications for loading strategies. **Strength and Conditioning Journal**. 36(2): 20-25, 2014.

OHTSUKI, T. Decrease in human voluntary isometric arm strength induced by simultaneous bilateral exertion. **Behavioural Brain Research**, 7(2): 165-178, 1983.

PAZ, GA; MAIA, MF; LIMA, VP; MIRANDA, H. Efeito do método agonista-antagonista comparado ao tradicional no volume e ativação muscular. **Revista Brasileira de Atividade Física e Saúde**. 19(1): 54-63, 2014.

PEREIRA, B; SOUZA JR., TP. **Compreendendo a barreira do rendimento físico**. São Paulo: Phorte, 2005.

POPE, ZK; WILLARDSON, JM; SCHOENFELD, BJ. Exercise and blood flow restriction. **Journal of Strength and Conditioning Research**. 27(10): 2914-2926, 2013.

ROBBINS, DW; YOUNG, WB; BEHM, DG; PAYNE, WR. Agonist-antagonist paired set resistance training: a brief review. **Journal of Strength and Conditioning Research**. 27(10): 2873-2882, 2010.

ROIG, M; O'BRIEN, K; KIRK, G; MURRAY, R; MCKINNON, P; SHADGAN, B; REID, WD. The effects of eccentric versus concentric resistance training on muscle strength and mass in healthy adults: a systematic review with meta-analysis. **British Journal of Sports Medicine**. 43(8): 556–568, 2009.

SCHOENFELD, BJ. The mechanisms of muscle hypertrophy and their application to resistance training. **Journal of Strength and Conditioning Research**. 24(10): 2857-2872, 2010.

SCHOENFELD, BJ. The use of specialized training techniques to maximize muscle hypertrophy. **Strength and Conditioning Journal**. 33(4): 60-65, 2011.

SCHOENFELD, BJ. Is there a minimum intensity threshold for resistance training-induced hypertrophic adaptations? **Sports Medicine**. 43(12): 1279-1288, 2013.

SCHOENFELD, BJ; PETERSON, MD; OGBORN, D; CONTRERAS, B; SONMEZ, GT. Effects of low- versus high-load resistance training on muscle strength and hypertrophy in well-trained men. **Journal of Strength and Conditioning Research**. Epub ahead of print, 2015.

SCOTT, BR; LOENNEKE, JP; SLATTERY, KM; DASCOMBE, BJ. Exercise with blood flow restriction: an update evidence-based approach for enhanced muscular development. **Sports Medicine**. 45(3): 313-325, 2015.

SIMÃO, R; DE SALLES, BF; FIGUEIREDO, T; DIAS, I; WILLARDSON, JM. Exercise order in resistance training. **Sports Medicine**. 42(3): 251-265, 2012.

SOUZA JUNIOR, TP; FLECK, SJ; SIMÃO, R; DUBAS, JP; PEREIRA, B; PACHECO, EMB; SILVA, AC; OLIVEIRA, PR. Comparison between constant and decreasing rest intervals: influence on maximal strength and hypertrophy. **Journal of Strength and Conditioning Research**. 24(7): 1843–1850, 2010.

SOUZA JUNIOR, TP; WILLARDSON, JM; BLOOMER, R; LEITE, DL; FLECK, SJ; OLIVEIRA, PR; SIMÃO, R. Strength and hypertrophy responses to constant and decreasing rest intervals in trained men using creatine supplementation. **Journal of the International Society of Sports Nutrition**. 8(1):17, 2011.

TEIXEIRA, CVLS; GUEDES JR., DP. **Musculação desenvolvimento corporal global**. São Paulo: Phorte, 2009.

TEIXEIRA, CVLS; GUEDES JR., DP. **Musculação perguntas e respostas: as 50 dúvidas mais frequentes nas academias**. 2nd ed. São Paulo: Phorte, 2013.

UCHIDA, MC; AOKI, MS; NAVARRO, F; TESSUTTI, VD; BACURAU, RFP. Efeito de diferentes protocolos de treinamento de força sobre parâmetros morfofuncionais, hormonais e imunológicos. **Revista Brasileira de Medicina do Esporte**. 12(1): 21-26, 2006.

WEINECK, J. **Treinamento ideal**. 9th ed. Barueri: Manole, 2003.

WILMORE, JH; PARR, RB; GIRANDOLA, RN; WARD, P; VODAK, PA; BARSTOW, TJ; PIPES, TV; ROMERO, GT; LESLIE, P. Physiological alterations consequent to circuit weight training. **Medicine and Science in Sports**. 10(2): 79-84, 1978.

WILSON, JM; LOWERY RP; JOY, JM; LOENNEKE, JP; NAIMO MA. Practical blood flow restriction training increases acute determinants of hypertrophy without increasing indices of muscle damage. **Journal of Strength and Conditioning Research**. 27(11): 3068-3075, 2013.

ABOUT THE AUTHOR

Cauê Vazquez La Scala Teixeira was born in Santos on the coast of the state of São Paulo, Brazil. In Santos, he graduated in Physical Education (UNIMES), he specialized in Physiology of Exercise (CEFE/UNIMES) and in Strength Training (UNISANTA), and obtained a Master's degree in Health Sciences (UNIFESP). He is a municipal public servant holding the position of Chief of the Section of Physical Evaluation and also acts in the segment of personal training. For some time, he has been sharing his practical activity between teaching and research at the Praia Grande College and at the Federal University of São Paulo, also participating as an invited professor in various specialization courses, university extension, congresses, and events throughout Brazil. His scientific contribution includes several books and scientific articles in the areas of weight and strength training, functional training, personal training, and physical evaluation. He was recently awarded the prize Top FIEP Brasil in the "book" (2012-2013) and "professional" (2013-2014) categories.

For further information, access www.caueteixeira.com.